~~(Number 1)~~

<u>HOW MANY TYPES OF VITAMINS ARE THERE?</u>

Apart from carbohydrates, proteins and fats in the daily diet, there are some other elements that are required by the body in small amounts. And due to lack of it, our body becomes diseased. Scientist Hopkins calls them "essential supporting food ingredients". In 1912, scientist Casimir Funk named the elements "vitamins".

<u>WHAT ARE VITAMINS?</u>

Although present in very small amounts in the normal diet, the dietary elements that boost our growth, nutrition and immunity are vitamins.

<u>PROPERTIES OF VITAMINS</u>

1. Our body needs it in very small amounts

2. Vitamins are organic catalysts in the body

3. Maximum vitamin acts as a co-enzyme in association with the stimulant.

4. Although most vitamins are damaged in metabolism, they do not affect digestion.

5. Plants produce most of the vitamins through synthesis, some vitamins such as vitamin A,
vitamin D, vitamin B-twelve, vitamin K, which are usually synthesized in the animal body.

6. Some vitamins are stored in the body.
Vitamin deficiency in the body is called avitaminosis in scientific language.

When our body has less vitamins than required, it is called hypovitaminosis.

VITAMINS STORED IN THE BODY

1. Pro Vitamins:

A pro vitamin is a vitamin that is synthesized from compounds. And those compounds are called pro-vitamins. The pro vitamin of vitamin A is beta carotene.

2. Anti Vitamins:

Compounds that interfere with the action of vitamins in our body are called anti-vitamins. Pyrithiamine acts as an anti-vitamin of vitamin B-1.

3. Pseudo vitamins:

The organic compounds in the animal body are complementary to vitamins, but not functionally equivalent to vitamins. Methylcobalamin, a pseudovitamin of vitamin B12.

SOURCES, FUNCTIONS AND DEFICIENCY DISEASES OF VITAMINS

VITAMIN A

Sources of Vitamins:

Both plants and animals produce these vitamins.
Plant sources: Cabbage, carrots, green vegetables, papaya, spinach, ripe mangoes etc. are vegetable sources of vitamins.

Animal Sources:

Liver secreted oils of some fish like heli bird, shark etc., egg yolk, milk, butter are animal sources of vitamins.

Functions of Vitamin A:

1. body growth

2. Rod cells in the retina of the eye protect us from night blindness.

3. Protects the infection of animal diseases.

4. Helps to maintain the normal function of the gland.

Deficiency symptoms:

1.Blindness is only caused by lack of vitamin A.

2. The skin of the human body becomes rough like the skin of a bang due to lack of vitamins.

3. Prevalence of weight loss.

4. Kidney stones are formed.

5. Power of infection is reduced.

VITAMIN B COMPLEX

Vitamin B complex is a combination of vitamin B-
one two, three, four, five, six and vitamin twelve.

SOURCES OF VITAMIN B COMPLEX:

Add a subPlant sources: Vitamin B complex is commonly found in abundance in red flour, green leafy vegetables, rice bran, tomatoes, yeast, sprouted chickpeas, etc.

Animal sources: Milk, butter, liver, egg yolk etc. are animal sources of vitamin B complex.

Functions of Vitamin B Complex:

1. Keeps the growth of the human body normal.

2. It helps in curing anemia, pleurisy etc.

3. Keeps nerve cells or brain steady.

Deficiency symptoms:

1. Beriberi is caused by vitamin B1 deficiency alone.

2. Diseases like tongue sores and mouth sores are caused by vitamin-B deficiency.

3. Vitamin B12 deficiency causes anemia.

4. In addition, lack of vitamin B complex causes hair loss, lack of appetite or nerve weakness.heading

VITAMIN C

Vegetable sources: All sour fruits like lemons, green chillies, tomatoes, amlaki etc. are rich in vitamin C.
Animal sources: Fish, meat, cow's milk and breast milk are found in excess of vitamin C.

Functions of Vitamin C:
----

1. Scurvy-preventing vitamin-C keeps gums healthy.

2. Role of vitamin C in red blood and platelet production.

3. Various mechanisms located in the body keep the work of reproduction under control.

4. Keeps the body healthy by healing wounds and preventing disease.

Symptoms of Vitamin C Deficiency:

1. Scurvy is only caused by vitamin C deficiency.

2. Anemia occurs.

3. Chronic diseases like bone and tooth decay mean vitamin C deficiency in the body.

VITAMIN D

Sources of Vitamins: Plant sources: Cabbage, carrots, green vegetables, papaya, spinach, ripe mangoes etc. are plant sources of vitamins.
Animal Sources: Liver secreted oils of some fish like heli bird, shark etc., egg yolk, milk, butter are animal sources of vitamins. In addition, vitamin D is produced by ultraviolet rays in the skin of the human body.

Functions of Vitamin D:
----

1. Helps in building bones in the body.

2. In short, calcium and phosphorus absorption, only vitamin D, does in the human body.

3. Causing the release of calcium in bones.

4. It helps in preventing rickets and osteomalacia.

Deficiency diseases:

1. Lack of this vitamin causes rickets in children and osteomalacia in adults.

2. Reduces blood calcium levels.

3. Lack of it causes caries or tooth decay

VITAMIN E

Plant sources: Green leafy vegetables, lettuce or sprouted chickpeas are sources of vitamin E.

Animal sources: Egg yolks, milk, butter are animal sources of vitamins.

Functions of Vitamin E:
----

1. Vitamin E helps in normal secretion of breast milk.

2. Removes blindness.

3. The uterus maintains the growth of the fetus.

4. Helps prevent miscarriage.

Deficiency diseases:
----

1. Deficiency of this vitamin slows down fertility.

2. May inhibit growth of the fetus in the uterus leading to death.

3. Breast milk production slows down.

VITAMIN K

Plant sources: Alfalfa greens, spinach, cabbage, tomatoes etc. are plant sources of vitamin K.

Animal sources: Milk, butter, liver, egg yolks are animal sources of vitamin-K.

Functions of Vitamin K:

1. Vitamin K plays a key role in preventing blood clotting in the body.

2. Keeps the amount of prothrombin in the blood natural.

Deficiency symptoms:

1. Deficiency of vitamin K occurs

2. Prothrombin in the blood, decreases.

VITAMIN P

Source of Vitamin P:

Vitamin P is very similar to vitamin C. Judging by the source of vitamin C, vitamin C supplements.

Functions of Vitamin p:

Vitamin p alone has no function of its own. This group of vitamins only helps to accelerate the action of vitamin C. And this is why its effectiveness and deficiency symptoms are similar to those of vitamin C.

SOME FOODS CONTAIN VITAMIN D

Your body needs vitamin D for calcium absorption and bone formation. When the amount of vitamin D in the body is reduced, children's bones are soft (rickets) and brittle, and adults have deformed bones (osteomalacia). You need vitamin D for other bodily functions.

Vitamin D deficiency has been linked to breast cancer, colon cancer, prostate cancer, heart disease, depression, weight gain, and other ailments.

Studies show that people with higher levels of vitamin D have a lower risk of developing the disease. However, it has not been proven definitively that vitamin D deficiency causes the disease – or that vitamin D supplements reduce the risk.

The Vitamin D Council – A scientist-led group raising awareness of vitamin D deficiency—they believe vitamin D treatment can prevent autism, treat autoimmune disease, cancer, chronic pain, depression, diabetes, heart disease, high blood pressure, flu, neuromuscular disease, and osteoporosis. may be helpful. However, human studies have not been conclusive.

The only proven benefit of vitamin D is that it helps calcium build strong bones. Vitamin D helps regulate immune and neuromuscular processes. Vitamin D also plays an important role in the life cycle of human cells.

Vitamin D is so important because our bodies make it themselves—but only if our skin is exposed to enough sunlight.ding

Dark skin absorbs less sunlight. That's why black people can't get enough vitamin D from sunlight like fair people.
Getting 30 minutes of sunlight on your face, legs, or back two days a week provides plenty of vitamin D.

Besides, vitamin D is found in egg yolk, cow's liver, milk, curd and cod liver oil.

Actually, vitamin-d is important for us because vitamin-d transports calcium to bones and makes our body grow very well! It also does many other tasks but this is considered the main task.

<u>**AND THE INGREDIENTS FROM WHICH WE GET VITAMIN-D
ARE:**</u>

1) Sunlight.

2) Various fish oils. For example: in cod fish oil.{{you can search about "which fishes contain vitamin-d" then you will find about this on Google. }}

3) Dairy/milk products.

4) Egg yolk etc.

Vitamin D is an essential vitamin that helps calcium function properly. Apart from this, it helps in keeping bones strong, skin healthy, hair healthy and mind healthy.

Sunlight is the main source of this vitamin. If you can apply the sun for 10-15 minutes in the morning, your body's need for this vitamin will be fulfilled. In addition, all milk and dairy products contain this vitamin - such as curd, yogurt, etc.

Better to say, 3 out of 5 women in their 30s and 1 in 5 men in their 40s are deficient. Lack of this leads to bone spurs and arthritis. So, don't forget to get it done once in a while along with various blood tests as per routine.

If you suffer from deficiency of this vitamin then do not panic at all. A 2 month course of injections or a course of medication can get you rid of it.

NOTE

(Number 3)

WHAT VITAMINS ARE IN ANY FOOD?

A vitamin is an essential biochemical component of food, which cannot be produced in the body and must be obtained from food. We think that vitamins give strength to the body, taking vitamins will reduce weakness or improve bad health - the idea is not correct. Vitamins do not produce any energy directly in the body. However, vitamins take part in the metabolism of different types of food, such as sugars, meats and fatty foods.
As a result, if one of the vitamins is lacking in the body, the activity of that particular element is hindered.
On the basis of biochemical properties, vitamins can generally be divided into water soluble and fat soluble. Fat soluble vitamins are A, D, E and K. Water soluble vitamins B and C. Water soluble vitamins do not accumulate much in the body.
As a result, if you don't take vitamin-rich food for a few days, it quickly becomes deficient. Fatty vitamins are stored in large amounts in the body for many days, so even if they are not taken in food for a few days, there is no problem easily.

Lack of vitamin A can cause night sweats, scaly skin, and decreased immunity. Deficiency of vitamin D causes clubfoot or rickets in children and osteomalacia in adults.

Vitamin K helps in blood clotting. Among the water-soluble vitamins, vitamin B complex is a combination of various vitamins. Their lack can cause beriberi disease, sores on the corners of the lips, anemia or anemia, reduced immunity, etc. A lack of vitamin C can lead to scurvy. All essential vitamins can be obtained through a balanced diet. Not all vitamins are found in the same food.

So all kinds of food should be eaten. Soluble vitamins are found in a variety of colorful vegetables, such as carrots, red cabbage, sweet pumpkin, fish oil, sprouted chickpeas, cabbage, spinach, cauliflower, etc. Sunlight is one of the sources of vitamin D. Water-soluble vitamins are available in milk, eggs, liver, i.e. animal meats, in addition to fresh fruits, vegetables, rolled rice. Sour fruits are rich in vitamin C. A variety of edible oils are sources of vitamin E. So vegetables should be cooked with little oil. There is no need to take extra vitamin pills if you take vitamins from the right food choices.

 Although vitamins and minerals are necessary for our body in small amounts, the deficiency of these food elements can lead to various fatal diseases. Based on solubility, vitamins are divided into two categories, water soluble and fat soluble. Vitamins B and C are water soluble and vitamins A, D, E and K are fat soluble.

Sources of Vitamin A:

Mango, cauliflower, carrot, tomato, pumpkin, sweet potato, liver etc.

Sources of Vitamin B:

Watermelon, eggs, milk, bananas, potatoes, fish, liver etc.

Sources of Vitamin C:

Mangoes, oranges, lemons, strawberries, various sour fruits, etc

Sources of Vitamin D:

Egg yolks, liver, mild sunlight etc.

Sources of Vitamin E:

Soybean oil, wheat, sunflower oil, cod fish etc.

Sources of Vitamin K:

Green vegetables, cauliflower, eggplant, liver etc.

<u>SOURCE OF MINERALS</u>

Potassium: Potatoes, cauliflower, green beans, carrots, bananas etc.

Calcium: Milk, yogurt, cheese etc.

Magnesium: Cauliflower, green beans, tomatoes etc.

Phosphorus: Fish, meat, milk, eggs etc.

Iron: Beef liver, cauliflower, green beans etc.

Zinc: Beef, cauliflower, green beans, tomatoes etc.

Iodine: Sea fish, salt, milk cheese etc.
Department of Gastroenterology

NOTE

<u>NO VITAMINS IN ANY FOOD</u>

Very good for eyes, hair and skin.

Some foods contain:
----

milk, carrots, sweet potatoes, sweet pumpkin, mangoes,
radishes, all green vegetables, cod liver oil, liver,
spinach, colorful vegetables, cheese, eggs, papaya,
beans.

Vitamin B

 Helps in proper digestion. Very beneficial for skin
 Some foods include: fish, any type of seafood, meat,
grains, eggs, dairy products, and green vegetables.

Vitamin C

 Helps to keep the various tissues of the body healthy.
Helps to speed up the healing process of the body. Increases immunity.
 Some foods contain: oranges, lemons,
strawberries, tomatoes, bell peppers, cauliflower, carrots, papayas,
pineapples, grapes, mangoes, yams, potatoes, watermelons, bananas, onions,
cherries, guavas, raisins, lettuce, eggplant, figs.

Vtamin D

 It is essential in the formation of teeth and bones.
 Very useful for strengthening teeth and bones.
It also helps the body absorb calcium.
 Some foods contain: milk, fish, egg yolks, liver.

Vitamin E

 Protects the lungs and helps build body tissue. Beneficial for skin and hair.
 Some foods contain: whole grains, green vegetables, egg yolks, various nuts,
sunflower oil, sweet potatoes, pumpkin seeds, palm oil.

Vitamin K

 It helps in blood clotting in case of a cut.
 Some foods contain: green vegetables, soybean oil, spinach, cabbage, lettuce,
mustard greens.

~~(Number 5)~~

<u>**WHAT IS THE PROBLEM WITH
ANY VITAMIN DEFICIENCY?**</u>

Lack of any nutrient causes the body to experience certain problems, sometimes physical, sometimes mental. This results in hair loss, various neurological problems, muscle spasms or pain, constipation and even mental depression due to lack of vitamins. Let's take a look at all the problems or symptoms that appear in the body due to lack of vitamins.

Let's take a look at the obvious.

If the skin is cut with a slight scratch or injury, it should be understood that there is a lack of vitamin C in the body. Besides, rough skin problems also occur. Sour foods can compensate for this vitamin C deficiency.

Dry or chapped lips are very common in winter. However, if the body is deficient in vitamin B12, this problem can occur in any season. Dandruff is a sign of fatty acid deficiency in the body. Also, lack of vitamin B (Vitamin B) hair becomes rough.

One of the reasons for premature graying of hair can be copper deficiency in the body. For this reason, you can eat foods containing copper such as cashews, mushrooms, etc. However, digestive problems or liver problems can also cause premature graying of the hair.

Lack of physical stimulation sometimes occurs despite adequate rest. Even after adequate rest, the body is tired throughout the day due to lack of vitamin D (Vitamin D).

However, apart from vitamin deficiency, the above-mentioned problems can occur due to various reasons. Therefore, buying vitamin supplements from the nearest drug store should not be consumed at all. Seek medical advice if necessary.

(Number 6)

VITAMIN AND MINERAL DEFICIENC Y DISEASES

We all know more or less that lack of vitamins and minerals makes the body sick. But none of us have a clear idea, exactly which vitamin and mineral deficiency causes which disease. We are more afraid of disease. If we know about these diseases, we can easily be alert and stay healthy. Deficiency of any vitamin causes any disease-heading

Vitamin A:
----
night blindness, xerophthalmia, degeneration of the cornea.
 Vitamin D:

Rickets in children, osteomalacia in adults
 Vitamin E:

Atrophy, megaloblastic anemia Vitamin K: Impairs blood clotting
 Vitamin C:

Scurvy, which causes swelling of the gums, bleeding and delayed healing of wounds.

Vitamin B1/Thiamine:

Beriberi is characterized by pain, swelling and watery discharge in the joints of the hands and feet.

 Vitamin B/2 Riboflavin:

Xylosis, Dermatitis, Glossitis Vitamin Niiasis : Plague Characteristic Weakness and special type of lesions on the skin of exposed parts of the body due to lack of Niiasis the skin of the hands becomes rough and red and turns dark.

 Vitamins Vitamin B6:

Mental confusion, nervousness Vitamin Biotis : Anemia, loss of appetite Vitamins Pentathenic acid : Burning foot syndrome Folic acid Macrocytic anemia.

 Vitamin B12:

Parnassium Anemia Vitamin Calcium: Rickets, osteoporosis Iron/Iron: Anemia causes deficiency anemia Iodine: Goitre, the symptoms of which are seen in the throat. Zinc : Loss of appetite, anemia Copper : Anemia Potassium : Weakness convulsions Magnesium : Muscle tremors, weakness and convulsions may occur. Fluorine: Dental Carriage Phosphorus: Preventing teeth and bone formation. Let us be aware of the above diseases. Our little awareness can keep us away from these diseases. Writer & Designer - Suvadra Rain Mondal

NOTE

(Number 7)

WHAT ARE VITAMINS AND WHY ARE THEY NEEDED?

Our body needs a very small amount of certain organic compounds for normal development and proper functioning of life processes; These are known as vitamins. Vitamins do not exactly provide calories or energy to our body, but ensure that we use the calories or energy we get from food in a good way.

Eating too many "processed" foods, staying up late, smoking, etc. increase our body's need for vitamins beyond normal. Also essential vitamins needed for a healthy body naturally. If vitamins and minerals are not in the right amount in the diet, it becomes difficult to keep the body healthy.

Vitamin A

Vitamin A increases the immunity of the body, keeps the eyes healthy. Lack of it causes loss of vision and many children even become blind. This vitamin is very important for the development of the body. To ensure the source of vitamin A in the body, aim to have more green, red and yellow foods in your daily diet. Vitamin A is available from beef liver, cod liver oil, egg yolk, milk, butter etc. The best time to take vitamin A is after exercise.

Vitamin K

Vitamin K helps in blood clotting. In addition, vitamin K plays a role in the secretion of bile from the gallbladder. This vitamin is usually made in the body. Vitamin K protects the body from osteoporosis. Vitamin K is available in food from green leafy vegetables, peas, green tea, oats etc.

Vitamin E

Vitamin E protects the heart, prevents skin aging, keeps muscles strong. If a food is cooked for a long time, the vitamin E in it is destroyed. The best sources of vitamin E are corn, soy, almonds, beans etc. Vitamin A is completely destroyed in fried, burnt or baked foods.

Vitamin C

Most fruits and vegetables contain vitamin C. However, most of the vitamin C is lost by cutting fruits or vegetables. Vitamin C prevents scurvy, heals wounds, nourishes red blood cells. A lot of vitamin C is available from amlaki, lemon, tomato, pineapple etc.

Vitamin B

Vitamin B or B complex is made by combining many vitamins together. Vitamin B is found in fresh fruits, vegetables, nuts, eggs, fish and cheese. Vitamin B aids in digestion, improves nerve function and prevents depression. Women can avoid "mood swings" by taking vitamin B before their period.

NOTE

Will taking vitamins increase energ

Vitamin is an essential biochemical component of food, which is not produced inside the body and must be taken from food. We believe that vitamins provide energy to the body, taking vitamins will reduce weakness or improve poor health. Actually the idea is not correct. Vitamins do not produce any energy directly in the body. However, vitamins take part in the metabolism of different types of food, such as sugars, meats and fatty foods. As a result, if one of the vitamins is lacking in the body, the activity of that specific element is hindered. Based on the biochemical properties, vitamins can generally be divided into water and fat-soluble vitamins. Fat-soluble vitamins are A, D, E, K.

Water-soluble vitamins B and C. Water-soluble vitamins do not accumulate much in the body. As a result, if you don't take this vitamin-rich food for a few days, it quickly becomes deficient. Fatty vitamins are accumulated in the body for a long time, so even if they are not taken in food for a few days, there is no problem. Lack of vitamin A can cause night sweats, dry skin, and immunity. Deficiency of vitamin D causes clubfoot or rickets in children and osteomalacia in adults. Vitamin K helps in blood clotting. Among the water-soluble vitamins, vitamin B complex is a combination of various vitamins. Their lack can cause beriberi disease, sores on the corners of the lips, anemia or anemia, decreased immunity, etc. Again, lack of vitamin C can cause scurvy.

All essential vitamins can be obtained through a balanced diet. Not all vitamins are found in the same food. So all kinds of food should be eaten. A variety of colorful vegetables, such as carrots, red cabbage, sweet pumpkin, fish oil, sprouted chickpeas, cabbage, spinach, cauliflower, etc., are high in fat-soluble vitamins. Sunlight is one of the sources of vitamin D. And in addition to fresh fruits, vegetables, rolled rice, milk, eggs, liver, i.e. animal meat, water-soluble vitamins are available in large quantities. Sour fruits are rich in vitamin C. And the sources of vitamin E are different types of edible oils. So vegetables should be cooked with little oil. Consuming vitamins through proper food choices will eliminate the need for additional vitamin pills.

NOTE

What are the types of
vitamin B complex

Vitamins are very necessary for our body, we all
know. And vitamins for the body are generally
divided into two categories. One is fat soluble
and the other is water soluble.

 Fat soluble vitamins include vitamins A, D, E and
K. All these vitamins can accumulate in our body
and they dissolve body fat. And water soluble
vitamins are B and C. They cannot accumulate in
the body but they dissolve water.

 If our body does not have a proper water
solution, then our urine will stop, the gum will
stop excreting from the body and various
complications will develop in the body.
Therefore, vitamin B is very important as a water
soluble vitamin.

 Vitamin B is the combined name of some
vitamins which is called vitamin B complex. You
may already know what vitamin B complex is and
why you need it. Now know its types.

 Vitamin B is not a single vitamin like other
vitamins, it is a group vitamin with 8 types of B
vitamins. Let's know about the different types of
vitamin B-

WHAT ARE THE TYPES OF VITAMIN B

There are 8 types of vitamin B and they are
----

*Vitamin B1 (Thiamine)
*Vitamin B2 (riboflavin)
*Vitamin B3 (Niacin)
*Vitamin B5 (pantothenic acid)
*Vitamin B6 (pyridoxine)
*Vitamin B7 (Biotin)
*Vitamin B9 (folate or folic acid)
*Vitamin B12 (cyanocobalamin)

Vitamin B1 (Thiamine)

Another name for this vitamin is thiamin, which works in the synthesis of sugars and amino acids in the production of enzymes for the body. Thiamine is very important for strong muscles and healthy nerves. Not only that, but vitamin B also works spontaneously for breaking down and digesting rice, bread, pasta, fruits and vegetables and storing the necessary solids from them.

A Dutch military physician named Christian Eikman discovered this vitamin in 1890. He originally discovered this vitamin while looking for the microbe responsible for beriberi. Christian Eikman discovered vitamin B1 while searching for the root cause of this difficult disease that leads to numbness of various parts of the body, difficulty breathing and sometimes death.

Vitamin B2 (riboflavin)

 Another name for vitamin B2 is riboflavin, which plays an important role in the formation of white blood cells. Vitamin B2 is also needed to provide energy to the body, maintain proper digestive function, and make vitamins B3 and B6 work.

 Riboflavin is very important for the body, it works to supply the necessary oxygen to all the organs of the body through the white blood cells.

Vitamin B3 (Niacin)

 The medical name of vitamin B3 is niacin, also known as niacinamide. This vitamin is needed to convert the carbohydrates and fats that come into the body with food intake into energy. In addition, vitamin B3 plays a special role in maintaining the health of the skin, the functioning of the nervous system and the proper management of the stomach. Deficiency of this vitamin causes three types of diseases, each beginning with D. These are dementia, diarrhea and dermatitis.

Vitamin B5 (pantothenic acid)

 Vitamin B5 is basically a type of acid that is necessary for the body called pantothenic acid. It helps the body absorb protein from a variety of foods, such as fish, meat, shellfish, and eggs. Even, vitamin B5 has a special role in the production of nutrients for the body by breaking down fats and carbohydrates.

Vitamin B6 (pyridoxine)

 Pyridoxine is an essential chemical for the body and is commonly known as vitamin B6. Pyridoxine is essential for the proper functioning of our nervous system. It also plays an important role in the production of important chemicals for our brain like serotonin. Vitamin B6 is most needed for mental health protection.

Vitamin B7 (Biotin)

 Biotin is a water-soluble B vitamin known as vitamin B7. Vitamin B7 or biotin is required for the proper metabolism of amino acids, cholesterol and some fatty acids necessary for the body. Vitamin B7 works more for healthy hair, glowing skin and healthy nails.

Vitamin B9 (folate or folic acid)

 Folate or folic acid is vitamin B9 that is commonly found in natural foods. Folic acid is very important for pregnant women to ensure proper conception. It plays a special role in the proper development of the unborn child, as well as helps in the formation of the nervous system and DNA of the unborn child. And we all know that there is no substitute for folic acid or vitamin B9 for the physical development and healthy life of the child.

Vitamin B12 (cyanocobalamin)

 Cyanocobalamin, commonly known as vitamin B12, is required for normal functioning of the human brain and nervous system. Vitamin B12 is essential to meet a variety of bodily needs, including the formation of white blood cells and the production of energy for the body.

 We learned more about vitamin B complex. I got an idea about what it is and how many types it is. Now for this vitamin needed by our body, we will eat those foods that have sufficient amount of vitamin B complex.

NOTE

~~Number 10~~

VITAMIN DEFICIENCY DISEASES
AND PROPERTIES OF VITAMINS

Hello friends how are you all? I know you are going through a lot of problems, right? See no matter how much we say we are not happy in our life. We may be needy even though we have everything. But many of us may not know or even try to know what that lack is. And those who have nothing are not in trouble but they are better off. Anyway friends today one very important thing that we always worry about ourselves or our parents or our children is good food or good vitamins. Vitamin deficiency or vitamin deficiency disease is the only cause of various problems of our people. We need to know the properties of vitamins.

Vitamins are biologically active substances that are active in many processes in the human body. Thanks to vitamins, we become happier, gain vitality and strength. More details about the properties of vitamins.

Vitamins have different chemical structures, but they have one effect – they help to release useful substances from products and additives. Vitamins help to regenerate and multiply body cells.
All vitamins have properties to increase immunity, reduce bad cholesterol levels, activate and enrich blood formation.
Vitamins also actively fight against aging, maintain the human body in a normal state, strengthen the process of tissue regeneration.

Functions and Importance of Vitamins

Vitamins:

Definition (Definition) – The special organic nutrient that helps the normal nutrition and growth of the body in very small amounts and increases the strength to prevent disease is called a vitamin.

Is vitamin deficiency dangerous

 If there is a lack of vitamins in the body, the metabolism slows down, the person's weakness, severe fatigue, headache, internal organ function may be disrupted. The nervous system is also damaged, and with it the immune system weakens.

 If the body is low in vitamin D, children may face depression, because there is not enough calcium left in the bones, they may not be strong and bend. The shape of the body also changes from this, the child can be very thin and thin hands and feet, they are weak, can not perform their functions.

 But if vitamin D is excessive, it has a negative effect on the body. Then the bone tissue, which contains calcium, transports it to other organs and receives nutrients from the heart, kidneys, intestines, and liver. From this, the functions of the internal organs are violated, they do not work well and the person becomes very sick.

 Feature of Vitamins:
----

 1. Chemical nature: Vitamin is a type of organic catalyst.

 2. Nature of Action: The vitamin acts in small concentrations and requires small doses daily.

 3. Sources: The main sources of vitamins are plants. However, vitamins A, D, B12, KA, D, B12, K are synthesized in the animal body.

 4. Other properties- (1) Vitamins are not destroyed by decomposition, but are destroyed during metabolism. (2) Vitamin acts as a co-stimulatory agent.

Importance of Vitamin
----

1. In normal growth: Vitamins are essential for the normal growth of the organism.

2. Prevention of diseases: The main function of vitamins is to prevent diseases.

3. Food as Prana: Vitamins are the essential food constituents for sustaining life of living organisms hence it is called as food prana.

Disease Name and Vitamin Name:

Toad-Skin or Phrynoderma – Vitamin A

Night blindness or Xerophthalmia – Vitamin A

Keratomalacia – Vitamin A

Renal Stones – Vitamin A

Beriberi – Vitamin B1B1

Pernicious Anemia – Vitamin B12B12

Pellagra – Vitamin B5B5

Stomatitis – Vitamin B2B2

Last words:

Vitamins are very necessary for ourselves or for our own physical abilities. So I will say one thing, don't let your own vitamin deficiency or your son's lack of vitamin.

NOTE

(Number
11)

VITAMIN K IN 5 FOODS

Everyone is more or less aware of the importance of vitamin K. This vitamin helps in blood clotting in case of bleeding. It also helps in bone formation. Vitamin K stores excess glucose in the body as glycogen in the liver and inhibits the formation of cancer cells.

Experts in the United States say that vitamin K is an essential fat-soluble vitamin. It keeps bones and heart healthy. Apart from this, it has many other needs in our body. You can easily get this vitamin in some vegetables that are easily available in the market today. According to the US National Institutes of Health, women need 122 micrograms of vitamin K per day and men need 138 micrograms of vitamin K per day. This amount of vitamin K can be obtained from vegetables that are easily available in the market. Here are some easy sources of vitamin K:

Turnip

Turnip is known as a winter vegetable. It is a kind of transformed root and underground part used as food. Half a cup of cooked turnips contains 426 micrograms of vitamin K. It has many disease-fighting properties. It is anti-inflammatory. It even helps fight cancer. It keeps hair and skin healthy. Eliminates anemia. It can remove bad cholesterol. Turnip helps to increase the immune system of the body. Its lutein content is beneficial for the heart. Since turnip is rich in fiber, it cures constipation. Turnip purifies the blood and helps in the growth of blood cells. Turnips are also very useful in reducing appetite.

Broccoli

 You can get 110 micrograms of vitamin K from half a cup of cooked broccoli. Nutritionists call broccoli a super nutritious vegetable. It has some great beneficial ingredients, which can prevent rapid aging. It is rich in vitamin C. Broccoli is ranked as the 10th anti-cancer food in the list of the American Cancer Research Institute. According to nutritionists, broccoli is rich in iron. A good source of Vitamin A. Also it is good for skin. Helps reduce cholesterol. It has a lot of antioxidants. It contains a lot of calcium. Helps to eliminate waste products from the body.

Carrot juice
----

 6 ounces of carrot juice contains 28 micrograms of vitamin K. Researchers say that drinking a glass of carrot juice every morning increases immunity. The most important benefit of carrots is to improve eyesight. Apart from this, there are many other health benefits. Works against harmful bacteria, viruses and various types of inflammation in the body. Apart from vitamins, carrot juice also contains various minerals, potassium, phosphorus, etc., which help in bone formation, strengthening the nervous system and increasing brain power.

Currant juice

There are 19 micrograms of vitamin K per six-ounce serving. Currants contain a lot of iron, potassium. Increases hemoglobin content. One mug of currant juice can be consumed daily to maintain hemoglobin levels. According to nutritionist Aleya Mawla, the fruit is not only beautiful to look at, but also unique in its nutritional value. It contains many minerals. So good for those who have anemia. Apart from this, there are a lot of nutrients such as amino acids, folic acid, potassium, antioxidants, vitamins A, C, E etc.

spinach

Eating cooked spinach increases the immunity of the body. It is a good source of vitamin K. There are many benefits of eating spinach. Spinach is rich in vitamin C and beta carotene which protects the cells of the colon. Spinach is very effective in improving memory and brain function. Spinach is a winter vegetable. It contains a lot of vitamin C. Source: Prevention.com, NDTV.

NOTE